The Smart & Easy Guide To Natural Remedies & Natural Therapy: How To Use Natural & Organic Healing Solutions To Reduce Stress, Improve Health, Slow Aging, & Get Better Nutrition For Women

Elizabeth White

Legal Stuff

COPYRIGHT

DISCLAIMER

THIS BOOK IS NOT DESIGNED TO, AND DOES NOT, PROVIDE MEDICAL ADVICE. ALL CONTENT ("CONTENT"), INCLUDING TEXT, GRAPHICS, IMAGES AND INFORMATION AVAILABLE IN OR THROUGH THIS BOOK ARE FOR GENERAL INFORMATIONAL PURPOSES ONLY.

THE CONTENT IS NOT INTENDED TO BE A SUBSTITUTE FOR PROFESSIONAL MEDICAL ADVICE, DIAGNOSIS OR TREATMENT. NEVER DISREGARD PROFESSIONAL MEDICAL ADVICE, OR DELAY IN SEEKING IT, BECAUSE OF SOMETHING YOU HAVE READ ON THIS BOOK. NEVER RELY ON INFORMATION ON THIS BOOK IN PLACE OF SEEKING PROFESSIONAL MEDICAL ADVICE.

THE AUTHOR, PUBLISHER AND ALL AFFILIATED PARTIES ARE NOT RESPONSIBLE OR LIABLE FOR ANY ADVICE, COURSE OF TREATMENT, DIAGNOSIS OR ANY OTHER INFORMATION, SERVICES OR PRODUCTS THAT YOU OBTAIN THROUGH THIS SITE. YOU ARE ENCOURAGED TO CONFER WITH YOUR DOCTOR WITH REGARD TO INFORMATION CONTAINED IN OR THROUGH THIS BOOK. AFTER READING THIS BOOK, YOU ARE ENCOURAGED TO REVIEW THE INFORMATION CAREFULLY WITH YOUR PROFESSIONAL HEALTHCARE PROVIDER.

LIMITATION OF LIABILITY

Table of Contents

Reducing Stress through Improved Breathing

Stress can be greatly reduced through meditation and proper breathing techniques. Improved and focused breathing coupled with meditation enhances relaxation, provides a sense of well being, ends mind chatter and has a calming effect that allows a person to feel more peaceful and emotionally centered.

Most formal religions and spiritual beliefs include some component of meditation. It can be argued that prayer itself is a form of meditation. Many forms of meditation, including yoga, are common elements found in the Hindu religion. Buddhist enlightenment is achieved through meditation and Jewish prayer also has a meditative component. In Christianity, prayer itself and the use of traditional prayer aids, such as rosary beads, are linked to meditation.

However, it should be noted that meditation does not need to be connected to religion or a spiritual belief. It can be used by anyone to reduce stress and anxiety and create balance among the physical, mental and emotional aspects of their daily life.

No special equipment is needed for meditation: all that is truly needed is a quiet place free of distractions. While some people prefer to sit in the lotus position while meditating – sitting with the back straight and legs crossed so that the feet are resting on the opposite leg's thigh – it is more important to be seated in a way that is comfortable for you. It is important to not be distracted by physical discomfort when meditating. Some people prefer to sit on the floor, but a chair can also be used.

When preparing to meditate, the most important aspect regarding posture is that the spine is straight and shoulders are not slouched. This keeps the chest and airways open, which facilitates deep, slow breathing and enhances circulation. Once seated comfortably and properly positioned in a quiet space, meditation can begin. Some practitioners prefer to remain quiet during meditation while others hum or repeat the word "ohm", letting sound resonate from the throat through the head. Many practitioners find that vocalizing in this way focuses attention inwardly and blocks outer distractions.

Meditation techniques can be used to help reach a relaxed, stress-free state of mind. One method has the practitioner focus on various parts of the body, one at a time, "asking" that body part to relax while deeply inhaling and exhaling. These are called "cleansing breaths" because they are intended to clear the mind of extraneous thoughts while delivering more oxygen to the internal organs and bloodstream. Continue breathing, focusing on a count of four during intake of breath and a count of eight during exhalation.

Since meditation is completely natural and enhances well being, it can be used as often as desired and needed. Unlike medication, which can have detrimental effects on the body over time and if overused, meditation can only improve your breathing and your life through stress reduction. While planned meditation sessions are often geared to last 20 to 30 minutes, you can use meditation anytime. Reduce anxiety quickly by focusing on deep breathing even for just a moment or two throughout the day as the need arises.

Research shows that meditation is quantitatively successful in reducing indicators of stress, such as blood pressure and heart rate; it also has been show to increase brain wave activity associated with calm, well being and euphoria. While pharmaceutical medications can reduce stress temporarily, they come with side effects that can cause more harm than good, especially when used for long periods of time.

Meditation is free of such side effects and can be used as often as desired; it is routinely used to improve the health of patients with chronic and terminal diseases. This is significant because there is a proven correlation between illness, poor health and stress. University of Colorado neurophysiologist, Dr James Austin, reported in 1999 that meditation actually reprograms the circuitry of the brain; these studies were further documented through the use of imaging techniques that map brain wave activity.

In addition, the Mind-Body Institute, which is affiliated with such prestigious institutions as the Harvard Medical Hospital, has reported that mediation actually results in physical and biochemical changes in the body that are linked to stress reduction: these include improved heart rate and blood pressure, more efficient respiration and metabolism, and positive changes in brain chemistry.

With such affirmative endorsements of the benefits of meditation and the ease of access for anyone to practice these techniques, one can readily see why more and more people are using meditation techniques to safely reduce stress and improve their health.

5 Basic Breathing Techniques to Reduce Stress

Since humankind's earliest days on earth, stress has been a part of life. When humans feel threatened or feel stress they automatically slip into the "fight-or-flight" response; that is we react to stress by fighting or fleeing. When we feel stress our bodies have a physiological response: heart rate and blood pressure rise; adrenaline and stress hormones kick into gear and our respiration levels increase. When you feel your body reacting to stress in this way, you can counter and reduce stress by practicing good breathing techniques. Breathing deeply allows for detoxification of the body and life itself. Without oxygen, our organs cannot properly function, resulting in illness and eventually, death.

When oxygen enters the body, it cleanses the blood of toxins; if we do not breathe properly this process is impaired and toxins build in the blood and organs. This toxic buildup can cause digestion issues, physical exhaustion and chronic anxiety, leading to a host of other physical, mental and emotional illnesses. It can result in failing health and an inability to cope with everyday life challenges.

Maintaining a healthy breathing pattern can reduce the effects of stress on the body; however, in order to learn breathing techniques designed to reduce stress, you first need to learn and practice basic breathing. Start by lying down on a bed, couch or the floor and get comfortable by letting your feet fall open; keep your legs about hip's width apart. Let your arms rest flat away from your body with your palms facing up and close your eyes.

Concentrate on breathing through your nose instead of your mouth; nasal breathing has more detoxification benefits. As you inhale, be conscious of your lungs and midsection filling with air and moving in unison. Exhale, and feel the air leaving your body as your lungs, chest and stomach collapse. Practice often this until it becomes second nature to you; this is the basis for the five stress relief breathing techniques.

The first technique is learning how to breathe deeply during relaxation. It can be done in any position, but is best done while lying down on your back. Bend your knees at a comfortable angle, keeping your feet about eight inches apart; turn your toes outward so that each foot points away from the other and keep your back perfectly straight.

Place one hand on the area just above your waist and place the other on your chest. As you inhale through the nose, breathe deeply so that the hand on your stomach rises as high as possible. The other hand, on your chest, should hardly move at all and it should move in unison with the lower hand. Continue with the process until it starts to feel natural. Next, you will try to smile as you inhale through the nose and exhale through the mouth.

While exhaling through the mouth, you should hear a slight sound, much like a breeze gently rustling the leaves of a tree. Pay attention to the sounds and movement of your body. Start out by doing this exercise for five minutes at a time and gradually build up to twenty minutes. When you finish each section, relax and be still for a few minutes before going on with your day.

A technique known as the "cleansing sigh" is another quick breathing technique that will reduce stress. Start in a seated or standing position, with a straight back and shoulders. Inhale as deeply as possible and then exhale with an audible sigh, as much as you can muster. Your next inhalation should feel automatic and natural. This technique can be done in repetitions of five through fifteen.

The next exercise will stimulate your nervous and circulatory systems while also reducing stress. Start out by standing up as straight as possible and extend your arms directly out in front of you, palms up. As you inhale, bend your arms at the elbows, bringing your hands toward your shoulders keeping your fists clenched. Exhale, keeping your fists tightly closed, as you push your arms out to extend in front of your body again. Do this exercise quickly ten to fifteen times in a row.

The fourth technique is known as suggestive breathing. Lie down and place both of your hands in the area between your ribs and stomach and take a few deep breaths. Concentrate on the intake of breath and imagine that it is being held right where your hands are place. As you exhale, imagine that oxygen rushing throughout your entire body. Do this exercise for five to ten minutes daily.

The fifth and final technique is called rolling breath. For this technique, you will need to enlist the help of a partner. Lie down and have your partner place one hand on your chest and the other on your abdomen. As you inhale deeply, imagine that your partner's hands are filling with air, starting from your chest and working down to your abdomen. Watch your partner's hands rise and fall with each inhalation and exhalation as you deeply take air in and out of your body.

All of these five techniques will help you both cope with and prevent stress.

Using Massage to Relieve Stress: Five Quick Techniques that work Magic

Massage is perhaps the most natural and instinctive way to heal ourselves. When we have a sore leg or tight shoulders, we naturally rub and knead the area with our hands to make it feel better. Massage is an excellent therapy for good health and stress reduction and can be used to relieve body aches and tension and it results in improved circulation, flexibility and improved sleep.

Massage is simply physical manipulation of the muscles and joints to relieve tension and stress in the body. Massage is based on human touch and without this kind of touch people can become depressed. Infants, who are not touched often, tend to have health issues and develop more slowly than infants who are frequently and tenderly touched. It has been shown that touching families raise children who are happier and healthier than those from non-touching families. Our society, however, has placed many taboos around the concept of touching; as a result, many people are conditioned to avoid it because they associate it with love and sexual behavior. Massage is about healthy, positive touch and eliminates taboos related to it. Here are five self-massage techniques that you can begin to practice right away so that you can enjoy the positive benefits of healthy touch.

Self-message is easily practiced on the shoulders and this is an area where many people experience a good deal of stiffness and pain. Shoulder pain can contribute to stiffness and tenderness in the neck; it also contributes to headaches and can lead to less than ideal posture. Begin your self-massage by using your right hand to gently knead your left shoulder. Start at the base of your skull and gently work downward along the neck, moving outward across the shoulder and toward your left hand. Work the area along your neck at least four times.

Now switch and use your left hand to do the right shoulder. Next, use your fingers to make circular motions up and down the neck and the base of the skull. Squeeze and release the areas around the shoulders and upper arms and gently tap along your shoulders with your fist. Do one side and then the other. Finish by using one hand to stroke the other, and then gently massage your face, chin, neck and shoulders one more time. This is an excellent massage when you need quick stress relief, especially if working at a desk or computer, as this tends to create stiffness in the neck and shoulders.

A leg massage is also very easy to do and it can help energize you and reduce fatigue after exercise or daily activities. Start by resting your foot flat on the floor. Starting at your foot, stroke your leg from bottom to top on both sides; repeat three times for each leg.

Next, work on your thighs: Doing this regularly can help maintain good muscle tone and skin texture. Use your fists to gently hammer each thigh; then massage the fronts and back of your knees. Make circular motions around the kneecaps using your fingers. Then knead your calf muscles and finish up by lightly stroking your calf muscles.

A foot massage is one of life's simple pleasures and while we all enjoy having a partner do this for us, it is very easy to give yourself a foot massage. Place your hands so that one is on top of your foot and the other is underneath; stroke your entire foot several times and then begin massaging each toe. Grab each toe individually, gently kneading and squeezing it. Using your fingers, rub the ball and the arch of the foot in a circular fashion. Then use your knuckles to massage then entire foot with circular motions. Stoke and rub the ankle and the entire foot, top and bottom.

A hand massage is also a great stress reducer and is very easy to do. It's a great remedy for hands that are overworked from garden chores or from overtaxing those muscles in any way. Start by stoking and then gently squeeze each part of the hand. Squeeze and massage each finger individually; make firm circular motions over the joints and then use the thumb of one hand to rub the tendons on the backside of your hand. Focus on the palm and make circular motions on it as well. Finish the massage by opening and closing your hand repeatedly a few times.

An abdominal massage is also easy to self-administer; it has the extra benefit of improving digestion and aiding in weight loss. Use your fingertips to knead the waist from one starting at one side and working across to the other. Use your hands to knead the area just above the hip bones and then work one hand across the abdomen in one direction, and follow in the opposite with the other hand. Repeat this sequence about ten times.

Self-massage is an easy way to relieve stress and improve circulation, and unlike going to a certified massage therapist, self-massage is totally free.

Food Choices: Why Organic is Worth it

People are more informed than ever about how food choices impact their health, for better and for worse and many people consciously make healthier choices than even just a few years ago. Since people are tuned into healthier eating choices, organically grown food is more readily available: Instead of having to go to specialty stores, you can find organic food in ordinary supermarkets and at your local farmer's market. Farmers who choose to farm organically, rather than using chemical fertilizers and pesticides, are not causing harm to our fragile ecosystem. Food that is free of pesticides and chemicals is better for your body as well.

Here are Five Reasons why organic food is worth the slightly extra cost:
1. Because they are pesticide and additive-free, organic food taste better, with a flavor that nature intended.
2. Organic food reduces use and reliance on non-renewable natural resources.
3. Organic food production is better for the land and protects groundwater, since it does not generate chemical or pesticide run-off into lakes, streams and rivers.
4. Organic farmers are also often small family run farms; buying their food helps save family farms.
5. Organic food is safe for children because it is free of additives, pesticides and chemical residues.

While organic food is typically priced higher than non-organic, think about how this difference can benefit your family. The avoidance of pesticides, chemical and additives can have a significant positive impact on overall health, especially over the course of a lifetime. People have become more aware of what goes into our food supply because of our access to information through the Internet and from endless media outlets. As a result, many people feel that the health benefits far outweigh the higher price of organic produce and foods. You can find many organic options in fruits and vegetables, as well as organic dairy and meat products, fish, bread, nuts, processed foods and baby foods in the organic section of your favorite store.

The word "organic", when applied to food, refers to the way that the food is grown and processed. Organic food is dependent on good stewardship of the soil that produces the food; compost and hydroponic methods are used to boost organic produce yields. Compost is a natural fertilizer, unlike synthetic chemical fertilizers that are sprayed on food to encourage large yields. The used of synthetic fertilizers and pesticides are prohibited in organic farming.

In meat and dairy production, the label "organic" means that no antibiotics are used to keep animals healthy. GMOs (genetically modified organisms) are prohibited in the production of organic food.

There are three categories of organic food labeling permitted by the US Department of Agriculture:
1. 100% Organic: This means that the item is made produced using 100% organic ingredients and/or growing methods.
2. Organic Made: This indicates food made of at least 95% organic ingredients; the remaining 5% is greatly restricted. In this category, GMOs are also prohibited.

3. Made with Organic Ingredients: This means that the food contains at least 70% organic ingredients and the remaining 30% is greatly restricted. No GMOs are permitted under this labeling category.

In order for the USDA to label a food as "organic", it must have a minimum of 95% organic ingredients. If a food has less than 70% organic content, it cannot use the word "organic" in any labeling or packaging. However, the producer is permitted to list specific ingredients that were organically grown on the ingredient label.

There are plenty of producers of organic food, both in terms of produce, dairy, meat and package foods. However, many people shy away from organic because the price is higher. Keep in mind that the price of organic food has been coming down and will continue to come down as more organic products become available; the greater supply of organic food makes the pricing more competitive. You should also keep in mind that buying organic food is like making an investment in your health and that of your family. While income may dictate what is affordable, keep in mind that some of the most reasonably priced organic food may be found at your local farmers market or farm stand. Growing a vegetable garden during warm weather months is great way to make organic food affordable for your family.

How to Naturally Combat the Depths of Depression

Depression is a growing concern in America. In their lifetime, one out of eight Americans will face serious depression; depression and related mood disorders affect approximately 25% of the US population. Depression can seriously impair one's ability to deal with day to day challenges and it can have a major negative impact on quality of life; so much so, that it is the leading cause of suicide. There are times in life when depression is a normal experience, such as when a person must deal with death, divorce or life changing events. However, depression becomes serious when it is prolonged and when a person starts contemplating suicide as a way to relieve emotional pain.

There are many causes of depression. Poor nutrition is one cause. If people have inadequate food or if they eat large amounts of processed food, they can fall short on needed nutrients that are necessary for proper bodily functions; this can have an impact on the brain and nervous systems. Some people also have toxic reactions to additives in food; things like pesticide residues and sugar substitutes, which are chemical cocktails, can be major triggers for depression in some people.

Depression can also be caused by food allergies; people with wheat allergies, in particular, seem to be prone to depression after consuming products made with wheat. Hormonal changes have also been linked to depression. Toxins in the body, high levels of stress, poor nutrition, and inadequate exercise can trigger these changes. When such hormonal fluctuations take place, they can result in mood swings and interruptions in how the brain processes information.

Insomnia and chronic interrupted sleep can also result in depression. Most adults require eight to ten hours of undisturbed sleep in order to recuperate from daily stress and are prepared to properly function the next day. If we sleep too much or too little, natural sleep and body rhythms are disrupted, which leads to stress, which then leads to more disrupted sleep, resulting in depression and an inability to function at normal levels throughout the day.

Exercise is a great tool that can be used to fight depression. Exercise releases hormones known as endorphins, the "feel good" hormones, which help to elevate mood; serotonin is one such hormone. People who do not exercise regularly have a 30% higher likelihood to suffer from depression than people who do exercise. While a doctor is more likely to recommend a drug like Prozac to treat depression, such drugs can have serious side effects; and why take these drugs when something as simple as a daily walk or ride on a bike can treat depression naturally? An exercise routine does not have to come with an expensive gym membership. Simple activities that you enjoy, such as walking, tennis, biking, cross country skiing, yoga, dancing and running, can be part of a varied exercise routine that keeps you motivated and active. Try to exercise at least three days each week for a minimum of twenty minutes. This is the minimum level required to detoxify the body, keep the heart healthy and increase serotonin in the brain.

There are also natural herbal supplements that can be used to combat depression. St. John's Wort is one such supplement that has been shown to help decrease depression, stress, insomnia, poor self-image and anorexia. When taking any supplement, continue to exercise and eat well. Most of these take time to have an effect and always check with your doctor or pharmacist to make sure it is safe to take supplements, especially if you are already taking prescription medications, as some supplements can cause serious interactions.

Ginkgo biloba is a supplement that improves blood circulation; this is significant because it means more blood flows through the brain and this helps detoxify the body. A chemical compound know as 5-HTP is also useful in the treatment of depression: It helps increase levels of serotonin, which in turn raises endorphins and other neurotransmitters which helps the brain from entering depressive levels. 5-HTP occurs naturally in the body but supplements can restore this amino acid to proper levels.

Vitamin and mineral supplements can also be helpful in combating symptoms of depression. Deficient levels of Vitamin B6 can contribute to depression and low levels of folic acid can result in insomnia, postpartum depression, anxiety, fatigue, inability to think clearly and irritability. Low Vitamin C levels result in low levels of serotonin, which leads to depression. People with low levels of magnesium may experience restlessness, cramps, tics, memory loss and anxiety. Focusing on these supplements may naturally reverse depression.

Of course, supplements should not be used in place of a healthy, well balanced diet. Good nutrition is a basic requirement for good health and can greatly reduce feelings of depression and anxiety. Vegetables and fruits are especially important and you should aim to consume 2 ½ cups of vegetables each day and 2 cups of fruit. Choose from many varieties to be sure that you are getting adequate nutrients. An easy way to do this is to choose fruits and vegetables from the various color groups: green, yellow, red, orange, purple, etc. Also, be sure that at least half of your daily intake of grain products is from whole grains. Choose low-fat dairy products or vegan alternatives, such as almond milk or coconut milk. Meat products should be lean or choose vegetarian sources of protein such as nuts, beans, kale and quinoa. Fish is a great source of omega fatty acids, which help protect the heart, brain and circulatory system.

Eat healthy fats, such as avocados, coconut oil and olive oil, and restrict the quantity of saturated fat in your diet; calories that come from saturated fats should make up no more than 10% of your total caloric intake per day. Read labels and do everything possible to avoid hydrogenated fats and trans fats, which are found in products like margarine and processed foods. They are the worst fats you can eat. Avoiding processed food and eating fresh, whole foods as often as possible is an easy way to be sure that you are avoiding chemicals and refined food products that are harmful to your heart, arteries and overall health. Go for fruits, vegetables and whole grain products and protein sources that are as minimally processed as possible. If you consume alcohol, do so only in moderation.

Create a Personal Retreat to Reduce Stress

Modern society creates stresses unknown to humankind in previous eras: The endless onslaught of demands from work, family and social obligations, as well as non-stop information bombardment from media and the Internet, makes it seem as though we never get any downtime. All of this takes a toll on the body, causing our adrenal glands to work overtime, pumping out stress hormones like adrenaline. The problem is that because of non-stop stimulation and demands, these stress hormones are not released occasionally, as they were for our ancestors; instead they are released nearly non-stop for many people on a frequent basis. This affects the body in a negative way, causing a rise in heart rate and blood pressure. Under stress, it is difficult to focus, function productively and even digest the food that you eat, so your body is deprived of nutrients.

Exercise can help reverse this hormonal onslaught upon your body, but if you are working at a desk job or stuck in your car when stress is delivered, these hormonal responses may go unchecked. If possible, pull over or get up and walk around for a few minutes and practice some of the deep breathing techniques described above. It can also be helpful to create a retreat for yourself where you can go to unwind at the end of the day.

A personal retreat does not have to be a vacation home or an expensive trip. It can simply be a room in your home that is designed to help you decompress from daily life. Many people turn their bathroom into an at-home spa, just for this reason. While bathrooms still serve the same functions as in the past, new and affordable amenities make it easier than ever to add spa-like comforts. Pulsating showerheads, even inexpensive versions that can simply be switched out with your current model, provide an invigorating and relaxing massage. Walk in showers fitted with benches, steam saunas and multiple showerheads are personal spas that can be enjoyed alone or with your partner. Spa tubs with pulsating jets are another great option. Such updates for the bathroom can range from affordable to expensive, so it's easy to add a few options that fit your personal needs and budget.

You can also create the feeling of a personal spa in your bathroom with some simple inexpensive changes. For example, you can paint the walls a soothing shade of aqua blue or watery green, add candles and soft, thirsty towels and bath rugs to bring comfort and warmth to the space. Aromatherapy candles and potpourri will enhance your spa experience; bath salts and bath oils are also a great touch, as are bubble bath, scented soaps and bath gels. Try some soothing music from a smart phone or media player; just be sure to keep it away from the water. Add some inspiration with stencils or wall art and your spa will be ready to welcome you whenever you need it.

Another way to create a retreat is simply by turning your mind inward and meditating. The wonderful thing about meditation is that you can use it anytime and anywhere. People who are experienced at meditation can even practice it while engaged in ordinary daily tasks, but beginners need a quiet place to meditate and, of course, you should never mediate when driving or during other activities that need your full attention.

To begin meditation, find a quiet place free of distractions where you do not expect to be disturbed. Sit on a pillow on the floor or, if that is not comfortable for you, you can use a chair. If you wish to close your eyes make sure that there is enough light in the room to keep from dozing off; sleeping is not mediation. You need to turn your thoughts inward and sleeping will not allow you to be mindful of that.

The main thing to keep in mind when you start practicing mediation is that you need to let go of obligations and "to do" lists: Simply do nothing. Relax, focus on your breathing and let go of individual thoughts as they enter your mind. Focus on yourself and see your life as part of a connected circle of life; try to look at the big things that are truly important, not the little things that will mean nothing two weeks or six months from now. In the early stages of meditation, it is better to avoid using mantras since that will make it harder to focus on yourself in this way.

The Growing Trend of Aromatherapy in Work Environments

Since approximately the year 2000, there has been a new trend in work environments: employers and businesses have seen the benefit of using aromatherapy in offices and places of business. Studies have shown that aromatherapy in work environments reduces not just job-related stress, but illness as well; and it increases productivity.

Research shows that aromatherapy protects against infectious diseases, such as the common cold and flu, and it can enhance worker morale and improve mood. There is also evidence that aromatherapy in the workplace encourages positive thinking and helps employees think clearly and logically. As stress is reduced in the workplace through aromatherapy, employees work more efficiently, are happier and more productive.

Another benefit of aromatherapy in the workplace is that it can be used to purify the air: Anti-fungal, anti-bacterial and anti-viral aromatherapies help reduce airborne bacteria dispersed from heating and air conditioning systems. They also reduce airborne bacteria and viruses passed from one person to another, so they can reduce the amount sick leave taken by employees. This is especially helpful in overcrowded workspaces and schools.

Purifying aromatherapies also appear to ionize static electricity which is significant in office and workplaces that have a great deal of electronic equipment, such as copiers, computers and so on. The static electricity created by these machines over charge the atmosphere and increase stress, tension and aggression in employees.

Given the highly stressful world we live in, both in our professional lives and private lives, it behooves employers to create a more positive and pleasant work environment. If employees connect pleasant feeling to their work environment, not only will they be more productive, but their improved attitude will spill over and positively impact other employees, which further reduces stress and the stagnation, as well as potential aggression toward other employees or customers. Aromatherapy in work environments helps to combat the negative influence of stressors commonly found in work environments, such as computers and equipment, lack of sunlight, noise, endless demands and deadlines, poor lighting and uncomfortable conditions. Stress in the workplace can cause bad attitudes, headaches, irritability, defensiveness, aggression, fatigue, poor performance and inability to concentrate.

Employees benefit from aromatherapy because their work environment is more positive and pleasant. They feel less stress and therefore it is easier to concentrate and complete tasks more efficiently and with fewer errors. Employers may benefit because aromatherapy reduces sick leave, increases productivity and improves morale. When employees are productive, healthy and happy, they have a positive influence on fellow employees and reduced absenteeism reduces backlogs, which is less stress for everyone.

There are many convenient methods for introducing aromatherapy in the workplace. Candles are an easy option, if this meets safety standards. Sprays, potpourri, scented oils and dispensers that plug into an outlet that dispense aromatherapy solutions on a repeated basis are also easy to use in many offices and work environments. Local stores, malls and online web stores have many options to choose from. If you work in your own office or cubicle, you may be permitted to include these items in your work space.

When choosing fragrances consider the effect of each type: Packaging will typically list the effect that is created by a particular aromatherapy fragrance. Here are some of the most widely used aromatherapy fragrances and their related effects:

• Frankincense creates a feeling of being centered and steady; it rejuvenates both body and mind and helps lessen anxiety.
• Chamomile is well known for its ability to create calm and reduce stress. It also combats depression, anxiety and sleeplessness.
• Geranium also reduces anxiety, eases tension in the mind and body and helps create balance in mood and emotion.
• Lavender creates emotional balance by creating mental relaxation; it also enhances clarity of thought and dispels anger and fear.
• Marjoram offers relief from emotional upheaval, tension and stress and helps calm feelings of nervousness and anxiety; it is also used to treat insomnia.

Staying Naturally Healthy with Home Remedies

Years ago, before doctors could write a prescription for a pharmaceutical drug, they depended on home based remedies that had been handed down from one generation to the next. And common maladies were handled at home from experience that also was shared from the elders. For example, mothers and grandmothers knew that the best way to stop hiccups in a baby was to offer them a little sugar on a finger. The sucking motion needed to take the sugar will stop the hiccup spasms nearly every time. Other favorite hiccup remedies include scaring a person, sipping water from a glass while being upside down and holding your breath.

Cold sufferers knew that a hot shower or bath or a holding your head under a tented towel while running hot water in the sink relieves congestion. Vapor rubs, chicken soup, and a mixture of honey and lemon juice in water are other favorites for relief of cold symptoms. Headache cures abound as well: Exercise gets the circulation going, which will often cure a headache, so taking a brisk walk can often help. A hot bath can have a similar effect because it fosters relaxation and opens capillaries, also stimulating blood flow.

Many people do not realize that dehydration can cause headaches. Drinking eight to ten glasses of water each day can prevent and cure headaches for many sufferers without the need for pain medication. Homeopathic treatments like acupuncture, acupressure and aromatherapy are also useful in treating headaches. To try it out, massage the skin flap between your forefinger and thumb; this is one of the pressure points used by acupuncturists to treat headaches.

Resting in a darkened room can also relieve headaches; bright lights seem to make headaches worse, particularly migraines. Hot and cold compresses applied to the painful area can help; alternate from one to the other for best results. Hunger and the resultant drop in blood sugar can also cause headaches; but don't eat sugar-laden junk food. Complex carbs or protein is a better option. Gently rolling your shoulders back and forth and up and down and rolling your neck from side to side can also reduce tension headaches.

There are many home remedies that quell uncomfortable side effects felt during pregnancy. Nausea and morning sickness can be avoided by passing on foods that are fatty, fried and spicy. Food with strong aromas, such as coffee, garlic and onions can also promote nausea. If pregnant, try eating many small meals throughout the day instead of three larger meals and don't let your stomach go empty for long periods of time. Two or three plain soda crackers with a few sips of water in the morning can often keep morning sickness away; drink the water at room temperature. Eat what appeals to you and you are less likely to get nauseous or vomit. Acupuncture can also help: Sea bands worn just below the wrist where the tendons are visible can stave off nausea. Remember that morning sickness it typical in early pregnancy but often goes away on its own after the first trimester.

Heartburn, whether pregnant or not, responds to many of these same remedies. Wearing loose fitting clothing is also advantageous as it keeps gas and acid from building in the gut. Slippery elm powder dissolved in warm tea is an old home remedy that works for many people.

Many people suffer from painful arthritis; arthritis is basically inflammation of the joints. While there are over-the-counter and prescription medications that are made to reduce inflammation, ginger extract is a natural anti-inflammatory. It works by removing oxidizing agents from the body without the side effects that come with many drugs. Ginger extract is 100% natural and free of side effects. Willow has been used for centuries to relieve arthritis pain; the ancient Greeks used it by mashing the leaves and mixing it with wine, then applying it to the painful area.

Lifestyle changes can also relieve arthritis. Gentle, daily exercise that doesn't stress the joints helps to keep them lubricated without causing more inflammation: Swimming, yoga, tai chi and bicycling are good choices as long as you don't exercise too long at one time. Allow sufficient rest between workouts. Certain foods cause more inflammation and should be avoided or eliminated: These include red meat, dairy products, tomatoes and red wine. Eating plenty of fruits and vegetables and taking Vitamin C supplements is also helpful to your joints, and overall health.

Vitamins and Minerals that Slow Down the Aging Process

Getting older is no fun. If you look in the mirror and see your mother or father looking back at you and you can't help but feel a little depressed. We also seem to lose our energy and zest for life as we grow older. While there have been many theories on the biological causes for aging, the most current evidence is that decreasing hormone levels are the primary culprit. This is the basis for hormone replacement therapy: Hormone replacement adds vitality, youthfulness, increases libido and improves brain function. However, hormone replacement therapy (HRT) is very controversial and many people and doctors feel that the risks outweigh the benefits, especially if you already have other risk factors. While there are HRT drug therapies freely available, many people opt for more natural intervention.

Many women suffer from an imbalance of estrogen and progesterone as they near menopause and after menopause. Such an imbalance can result in weight gain or loss, fatigue and mood changes, hot flashes, depression and fuzzy thinking or memory loss. Soy products are often used to mimic estrogen in the body and are used to replace its function. Soy based creams that are absorbed through the skin have given many women relief from post-menopausal symptoms.

Free radicals are another threat to our health and the harmful effects of free radicals are cumulative, so the damage is more obvious as we get older. Free radicals are unstable molecules in our bodies that search for other molecules in our bodies to stabilize themselves, much as a proton and neutron seek out each other in a chemical reaction. When free radical molecules collide with other molecules in our bodies they actually emit a flash of light. Not all free radicals are bad: Some are beneficial in helping to reduce inflammation, fight off bacteria and control the smooth muscle tissue in your body.

Smooth muscle tissue is important in the regulation and functioning of the internal organs. The problem arises when there are too many free radicals in your body because they don't differentiate between healthy and unhealthy aspects of your body's make up. This kind of activity can result in heart disease, artery disease and cancer.

Chemical substances known as antioxidants have been found to be very helpful in combating the activity of free radicals. They can actually slow down or reverse the growth of cancer cells and can be considered to be anti-carcinogenic. Antioxidants work by giving away an electron to a free radical, rendering it neutral and safe. Antioxidants protect the membranes of blood vessels, the heart and the brain by neutralizing free radicals. Antioxidants are found in vitamins and minerals, particularly those found in fruits, vegetables and grains.

Here are some of the most important antioxidants:
• Carnosine is found in high quantities in the brain, as well as tissues of the muscle and those that make up the lens of a human eye. It protects the membranes of cells and the structures that make up the cells. It is useful in preventing muscle fatigue, improving sleep and reducing anxiety, hyperactivity and stress.

• Lycopene is found in tomatoes and it is important to replace this antioxidant because we tend to lose it as we age. Lycopene protects the digestive tract from cancer and is also helps protect the tissues and function of the adrenal and prostate glands, the liver and the testes.

• Lypoic acid is an antioxidant that also helps convert carbohydrates to energy. It works by destroying free radicals in the watery compartments of cells and prevents cell oxidation. It is also responsible for the breakdown of sugar so that the body can use it for energy. Lypoic acid is known as the universal antioxidant because it is soluble in both water and fat cells, so it is able to neutralize free radicals in either.

• Xanthones protect the nerves and nervous system with their strong antioxidant powers. It is bitter to the taste and can elicit feelings of euphoria. It is used to help patients battle depression and it can also be helpful in suppressing appetite and compulsive behaviors. Xanthone works by triggering hormonal reactions that ultimately release dopamine into the areas of the brain that detect and produce pleasure.

• Dopamine is a neurotransmitter that produces energy in the brain; it is capable of decreasing or increasing the output of brain cells. It stimulates activity in the brain and stimulates the pituitary gland, which in turn improves immunity to disease and stress and releases growth hormones. As we age, dopamine production decreases but blueberries have been found to be a good source of antioxidants that can reverse the effects of dopamine reduction.

The Benefits of Exercise: Quick, Effective Workouts for your Busy Life

We have long known that regular exercise can help people reach their fitness goals, but we also know that it can lead to better health as well. Exercise contributes to a long lifespan, helps to prevent disease, makes it easier to control body weight, and can help patients better manage chronic diseases like diabetes. Exercise also makes it easier to maintain good muscle tone, reduce fat and stay flexible. When we exercise, our heart rate increases, which improves circulation and keeps the arteries clear; this reduces the risk of developing a blood clot, which can result in stroke, heart attack or death. Staying active and engaged in regular physical fitness activities is like magic pill for maintaining a youthful appearance and it keeps the body at peak performance.

Fitness helps us perform at our best when working and meeting everyday obligations, and it gives enough excess energy to enjoy leisure activities when our work is done. Being fit allows you to perform at a level beyond what is expected on average from people in your same age group. Fitness is at the core of extraordinary health.

Fitness does not just affect your physical makeup, it also improves your mental outlook, emotional health and brain function. If you feel physically energized and strong, your mind will follow suit. While we all know that we should be exercising at least several times a week, many people have trouble finding time to fit exercise into their daily schedule. However, there are several mini-workout routines that you use to get more physically fit – and these don't take a lot of time.

This first routine will take about ten minutes, but you can lengthen it when you have time to do more. Start by walking for five minutes at a moderately brisk pace; be sure to pay attention to posture, staying as tall and erect as you can. Next, walk as fast as you can or jog for three minutes. Then do two more minutes at your original walking pace. As you become more fit and when you have more time, such as on the weekends, you can gradually extend the length of your workout.

People find that walking or a combination of walking and jogging is a good workout choice because anyone can do it and it does not require special equipment or a lot of prep time. All you really need is a good pair of walking shoes and a watch. If you have a smart phone, there are several free apps that will keep track of your daily walk, your pace and goals. Walking is relatively harmless as it does not overtax the joints. Another great benefit of walking is that it can be done anywhere and anytime, whether you are at home, on vacation or on a business trip.

One of the great benefits to walking is that it increases your energy and fitness level, clears you mind and lets you enjoy the great outdoors and fresh air. When you start a walking program, start at a pace that is a challenge but not so fast that you get shin splints or pain; choose a pace that you can maintain for the entire length of your walk. Many people find it easier to walk by time, rather than miles; for example, you may start out at 15 minutes per session and build up to an hour or more. If you start to feel pain or shortness of breath, slow down a bit and try to increase your pace again after a few more sessions.

This next workout will take approximately fifteen minutes. During the first two minutes, climb a flight of stairs repeatedly or do jumping jacks. Next, power walk for eight minutes, then repeat the stairs or jumping jacks for three more minutes. Finish with two minutes of walking at a brisk pace.

If you have twenty minutes to devote to a fitness routine, start out by stretching for two minutes: Stretch from one side to the other, reaching down toward your feet with your arms. Bend at the waist, keep the spine straight. Next, do a few minutes of squats with your hands in position, as if you are holding an imaginary barbell overhead. Now, jog in place for three minutes and then do a minute of lunges. Next, place your feet together and jump from side to side for one minute, followed by another minute doing as many push ups as you are able. For one minute, stay in a push up position but alternate bringing your knee up toward your hands; first the right side, then the left. Now repeat the whole sequence again and then spend one minute to cool down.

This next workout is geared toward building the upper part of the body and takes approximately ten minutes. Do step ups on a stable bench or step for one minute; then do wall pushups for one minute. The third minute is a shuffle exercise: Stand with your feet hip width apart and slide the left foot till it meets the right; spread the feet apart and again and continue the entire length of the room, as if your feet are joined with a rope. The next minute is spent doing pull ups to strengthen your upper body: Use a pull up bar that installs in a doorway; you can get one at a fitness store. You can also use a broomstick between two stable chairs; lie beneath it and pull yourself up for one minute. Do knee lifts for the next minute, alternating and lifting as high as possible and finish with one minute of concentration curls with a hand weight.

Workout five focuses on the lower body: Start again with a minute of step ups, followed by two minutes of lunges and then two minutes of the shuffle described above. Then do three minutes of running in place with your knees brought up as high and close to the chest as you can. Then finish with two minutes of stair running.

Workout six is for abdominal strength. Do two minutes of the following sit up: Lie down on your back on the floor and raise our arms up; roll up from the shoulders, through the neck and then the head. Repeat as many times as possible during the two minute session. Now do two minutes of the shuffle exercise followed by three minutes of running or jogging in place. Finish with three minutes of stair running.

The seventh ten-minute workout is easy to remember: Simply jump rope for ten minutes. This exercise can be done anywhere, anytime and is very good for maintaining strong bones. Workout eight is also easy to remember: It is ten minutes of squats and lunges with weights in each hand; this is a fast upper body workout.

The ninth and tenth workouts are also simple exercise regimens that can be done nearly anywhere: Number nine is simply running the stairs in your office or another building; or use outdoor stairs. The tenth workout is a good stress buster that will revitalize you during the work day: Do fifteen minutes of stretching, working on each part of your body. This will relax tight muscles, improve blood flow and banish afternoon fatigue.

Nutrition 101: Eating Right Made Simple

Weight control is about balancing calories: When you consistently burn more calories than you take in, you will lose weight. It's that simple. But, many people also need to be conscious of what they eat not just from the perspective of weight, but also so that they get proper nutrition. You have to fuel your body properly in order to maintain good health.

Eating "right" means a combination of things: You need to eat a variety of foods, limit or eliminate processed food, eat certain foods and beverages in moderation, and watch overall caloric intake. A well balanced diet does all of these things and as a result, it helps keep you healthy and physically fit; eating healthfully most of the time reduces the risk of developing high cholesterol, high blood pressure, heart disease and diabetes.

Our bodies function best when we consume the right balance of various nutrients. For example, carbohydrates (carbs) provide energy. Your body builds a supply of glucose from carbs and this store of glucose can be used immediately or stored for later use. However, if you take in too many carbs and are not active enough to burn them off relatively soon, they are stored as fat in your body. Carbohydrates are found in two forms: Simple and complex. Sugar is a simple carbohydrate and fibers and starches are complex carbs.

Protein, another critical nutrient, is responsible for the creation and maintenance of muscles and tissues. Protein is also important in hormone production and, just as with carbohydrates, excess protein is stored as fat by the body. There are two main sources of protein: animal and vegetable. Animal protein is higher in fat however, particularly saturated fat, which can lead to high cholesterol and heart disease.

While we have all been condition to avoid fat, there are actually healthy fats that your body needs in order to function properly. Fat can be saturated or unsaturated. Saturated fat is to be avoided; unsaturated fat, from foods like avocados, are healthy for you; however, if they are processed, unsaturated fats can become saturated and unhealthy.

To stay healthy, we also need to consume vitamins; each type of vitamin has a different function in the body. Vitamins are linked to metabolism and create energy; particular vitamins can also help prevent certain types of disease. For instance, Vitamins E, C and A are known as antioxidants. They help prevent cardiac and coronary artery diseases because they work to keep the insides of the arteries free of plaque. Plaque in the arteries can lead to clots, heart attacks and strokes. The B Vitamins are also very important: B-1 aids in digestion and supports the nervous system. B-2 helps with healthy cell growth and B-3 keeps toxins from building in the body. Folic acid, a B Vitamin, is essential in the creation of red blood cells. Vitamin D allows calcium to be absorbed by the body and Vitamin K is needed so that the blood can clot when you are injured or have surgery.

Your body also requires minerals and trace elements to perform various bodily functions. Phosphorus is related to strong bones and chlorine is needed to create digestive fluids that help break down food so that nutrients can be absorbed. Sodium is another essential nutrient: While we should limit our intake of salt to no more than 2400 milligrams daily, we do need some salt in our diets.

There are some basic guidelines that everyone should follow to get the nutrients you need each day.
• Eat at least 2 ½ cups of vegetables and 2 cups of fruit each day. Choose a variety from each group and each from each of the five subgroups of vegetables at least four times every week.
• Make at least half of your grain intake from whole grains. You should eat at least 3 ounces of whole grain products daily.
• Choose low fat dairy products or substitute non-dairy sources of calcium such as soymilk, soy cheese, coconut milk, or almond milk. The recommended intake of dairy or dairy substitutes is 48 ounces daily from low fat sources.
• Avoid saturated fat. Consume fats from unsaturated sources as much as possible. Saturated fats should make up no more than 10% of your total caloric intake each day. Avoid trans fats and hydrogenated fats entirely.
• Choose lean sources of protein including lean meats and poultry, fish, beans and legumes.
• Consume alcohol in moderation. Alcohol is mainly sugar but offers few nutrients, so these are essentially empty calories.

Good nutrition is the cornerstone of good health. While treats are okay occasionally, you should strive to eat nutritionally balanced meals and healthy foods at least 80% of the time and supplement your diet with a good multi-vitamin.

How a Macrobiotic Diet Can Improve Your Health

Those who practice macrobiotic dieting see the food we eat as having a direct correlation on not just physical health, but also emotional well being and overall satisfaction with life. Macrobiotic practitioners believe that food has a major influence on the quality of life and the quality of the food you eat is of paramount importance.

Macrobiotic practitioners believe that food that is in its most natural state is the most beneficial to the body. They shun processed foods but use traditional cooking methods. The word itself "macrobiotic" literally means "great life". Both philosophers and medical doctors have expanded the meaning to include "oneness" with nature; it is a simple and balanced diet based on food as nature intended. George Ohsawa coined the macrobiotic diet during the 1920's; he claimed that his serious illness was cured after switching to this type of diet.

Ohsawa based his study of macrobiotic diets on the Chinese philosophy of Yin and Yang. Yin and Yang are total opposites: one is black, the other white. One spins in an outward direction, while the other spins inward and both create centrifugal force. Yin is sweet, while Yang is salty. The dichotomies continue as one represents hot and the other, cold; passive versus antagonistic. Macrobiotic nutrition is based on this concept of push/pull: the diet must be kept in balance in order to maintain optimum health.

Various classes of foods fall under one or the other category based on their flavor, their properties and how they affect the body. Grains and vegetables are considered neutral in terms of yin-yang, so they are very important in creating balance against other foods that are extreme in terms of either set of characteristics. Foods that are extremely yin or yang are avoided.

Of course, pesticides, fertilizers and chemical additives have no place in a macrobiotic diet; so all food must be organically produced. The most balanced foods found in a macrobiotic diet are whole grains; whole grains like brown rice, millet, rye and whole wheat comprise the greatest portion of what is consumed. Whole grains fill about 50 to 60% of the diet. Bread and pasta are the least desirable of the grains but are acceptable in small amounts if they are made from whole-wheat flour.

Approximately 25 to 30% of the diet is made up of fresh vegetables. Those following the diet are to eat mostly from the following: cabbage, broccoli, kale, cauliflower, turnips, collard and mustard greens, radish, onion, acorn and butternut squash and pumpkin. Other vegetables such as lettuce and celery, snow peas, mushrooms and string beans can be eaten just twice or three times each week. The goal is to eat the vegetables as minimally processed as possible, so they can be eaten raw or lightly steamed; sautéing in unrefined cooking oil is also acceptable.

Sea vegetables and beans make up another 5 to 10% of the diet. The preferred varieties of beans are chickpeas, lentils and adzuki beans; tofu is also part of this portion of the diet. Sea vegetables are highly esteemed in the macrobiotic diet because they are so dense in nutrients and vitamins. Soups are an integral part of the diet, as well, and they make up approximately five to ten percent of total consumption: Soybean paste or miso should be included in the preparation of the soup, and beans and vegetables are also included.

Foods that are included on a limited basis (a few servings each week) include fresh fish and nuts. Sugar and mainstream sweeteners like honey, as well as artificial sweeteners are completely avoided; acceptable sweeteners include rice syrup and barley malt. Small amounts of brown rice vinegar and plum vinegar are occasionally used, as is sea salt and tamari soy sauce.

Beverages are not a priority in a macrobiotic diet and followers only drink when thirsty. Purified water and teas that are made from dandelion greens or roasted grains, or the water used to cook soba noodles are the only acceptable beverages. Coffee and teas that contain caffeine, flavorings or aromatic enhancements, such as herbal teas, are forbidden. All water that is used for cooking or drinking must be purified before using.

Foods that have preservatives or artificial colors or flavorings are forbidden in the diet as well. Foods with strong yang sensibilities include eggs and dairy foods. Chocolate, sugar and foods with sugar, coffee, fruit juice and soda, as well as hot spices fall under the yin category. All of these are avoided.

While the macrobiotic diet can seem foreign to someone unfamiliar with its tenets, many people who follow the diet report much improved health and vitality beyond their years. This basic, natural diet is as much a lifestyle choice as it is a way of eating.

How Acidophilus Can Make You Healthier

While we all know that bacteria can cause infections and be harmful, we need to remember that there are also "good bacteria" in the body. Lactobacillus acidophilus is in this group of good bacteria: Everyone has these friendly bacteria in their intestines; it is also present in women's vaginas. Lactobacillus acidophilus, also called simply acidophilus, is attracted to acid and it protects the body from organisms that can cause harm.

When acidophilus becomes depleted in the body, as a result of using products like contraceptive creams for women or when we take antibiotics, harmful bacteria and organisms can gain a foothold in the body and cause illness and disease. Therefore, it is important to replace these good bacteria when you use such products or antibiotic.

Acidophilus works by producing lactic acid and hydrogen peroxide, along with related byproducts when food is digested. In this way, acidophilus creates an environment that makes it difficult for harmful bacteria or organisms to exist. Acidophilus also consumes the nutrients that harmful bacteria thrive on, so this also slows down the growth of such pathogens and unhealthy organisms.

Acidophilus offers additional benefits that protect our bodies from stress and aging. It helps the body produce niacin, pyridoxine and folic acid during the digestive process, and it works to separate bile acids from amino acids. While this sounds complicated, the important thing to keep in mind is that these amino acids can then be recycled and used again by the body, which is like an insurance policy against the ravages caused by toxic substances like alcohol and drugs.

Acidophilus is added to yogurt and specialty milk products; look for it on the label of these products. It naturally occurs in many foods as well: bananas and carrots, soybeans, rice starch, garbanzo beans and garlic. It can also be purchased as a supplement in the vitamin aisle of your favorite stores and it is a good idea to take these supplements when you are on antibiotic therapy.

Some acidophilus products are also fortified with bifid bacteria, which is also good for digestion. Some contain other nutrients and vitamins and can be used as a good daily supplement. Acidophilus drinks have the best effect when taken on an empty stomach about one hour prior to meals.

Acidophilus has been shown to stop and prevent growth of Candida, which is a yeast or fungus that lives in moist, warm areas of the body, such as the intestines, mouth and genitals. When the growth of Candida gets out of control, it can form white patches in the mouth, known as thrush. If left unchecked, this infection can spread to the lungs, liver and skin. In the vagina, Candida can cause vaginal yeast infections, which result in burning, itching and painful intercourse. Diaper rash is another form of Candida; the skin becomes infected from Candida bacteria that are spread from feces to the skin. Candida infections are common in babies, children and people with depressed immune systems, so acidophilus supplements are very helpful in avoiding and clearing up these infections. Acidophilus powder can be added to baby formula once per day.

Women who have chronic and reoccurring vaginal yeast are able to clear and prevent future outbreaks by eating yogurt that contains acidophilus; the yogurt should be eaten daily to maintain a healthy bacteria balance. Additional research shows that acidophilus is useful in improved function of the gastrointestinal tract and in strengthening the immune system. Many people find it helpful in the treatment and control of diarrhea, indigestion and gas, and infections of the urinary tracts; it even helps to clear up acne and freshen breath.

Oklahoma State University completed a study of acidophilus and its effect on cholesterol levels: The study showed that acidophilus can reduce high levels of serum cholesterol and it also reduces the risk of heart attacks and coronary diseases for patients with high cholesterol.

Ten Teas with Healing Properties

Tea is not only fragrant and delicious; it is also very good for you. Tea is loaded with antioxidants that have been proven to slow the aging process and fight cancer cells. Some teas contain polyphones that improve digestion and reduce dental plaque, thereby helping to protect teeth; others have vitamin C to help ward off colds and flu.

The healing potential of tea is so great that you should make an effort to include tea as a beverage that you frequently enjoy. Here are ten tea therapies to tempt your taste buds and boost your health:

1. Green Tea: These are the most popular teas of Asia and include very popular varieties, such as Jasmine Green Tea, Green Peony Tea and Roasted Green Tea, but all varieties of green tea are high in antioxidants, minerals and nutrients. Once green tea is picked, hot air is used to dry it and then the leaves are pan fried. Green tea leaves are not fermented and this is why so many nutrients are retained. Vitamin C naturally occurs in green tea; this is why green tea supports the immune system. Green tea also naturally contains fluoride, which helps to prevent tooth decay and maintains strong bones.

2. Oolong Tea: This tea is known for its ability to calm indigestion and it also helps lower serum cholesterol levels in the blood. Oolong is made from the leaves of full-grown trees; they are picked and then left to air dry and partially ferment in the shade. This tea is naturally sweet and aromatic, with a pleasing aftertaste. Popular varieties include Jasmine Oolong Tea, Hairy Crab Oolong Tea and Ice Peak Oolong Tea.

3. White Tea: This mild tea is made from young, tender tea leaves that are still immature enough to be covered with silvery down. Instead of fermenting the leaves, they are steamed and then dried in sunlight. Since they are not fermented, white tea leaves are full of compounds that naturally combat cancer cells. White tea has a very fresh taste and pleasant aroma. Jasmine Silver Needle, White Peony and Silver Needle are very well known varieties.

4. Black Tea: These are the most common and popular teas of Western societies and are the basis for well known English teas. These leaves are picked and then fully fermented so that the leaves darken until they are nearly black. Black tea can have a variety of flavors, from overtones of fruit or flowers, to a spicy or nutty essence. Black tea is loaded with antioxidants and it is renowned for its ability to reduce tendencies toward blood clots, thereby reducing the risk of strokes. There are many popular varieties of black tea including Rose Black Tea, English Breakfast Tea and Earl Grey.

5. Chamomile Tea: Actually an herbal tea made from flowers in the daisy family, this mild, aromatic tea is popular for reducing muscle and menstrual cramps, reducing inflammation, and providing relief from toothaches. One of its most common uses is to provide relaxation and promote sleep.

6. Rosebud Tea: This tea is also made from flowers, specifically the rosebuds and rose hips of a shrub rose. As expected, sweet floral overtones are predominant in this tea and rosebud tea is often brewed in combination with other types of tea. Rosebud tea contains essential oils that help promote good circulation and rose hips are chock full of vitamin C, making this tea great for immune system support.

7. Wild Holy Tea: Used more for its curative powers rather than casual enjoyment, wild holy tea is bitter to the taste but has great detoxifying power. It also helps promote good circulation and digestion, and if consumed regularly, it is helpful in controlling blood pressure and body weight.

8. Milk Tea: This is one of the two most popular teas in Sri Lanka and India; the other favored tea of those regions is spiced Indian black tea. This tea is a concoction of milk and spices that brewed together; its rich flavor reveals cardamom spice, ginger and cinnamon. It is often blended with other types of tea as well.

9. Red Tea: This tea is growing in popularity and has a rich, nutty flavor. Red tea is grown in Africa. It is free of caffeine and also has a very high concentration of antioxidants; studies show it to be extremely useful for immune system building and support. Favorite varieties include Organic Cape Red Tea, Organic Green Summer Red Tea and Florida Orange Red Tea.

10. Paraguay Mate: This is one of the most popular teas of South America and it is typically served in a hollowed gourd with a straw. It is brewed with a variety of spices and is known for its ability to provide an energizing, combat depression and improve digestion.

Enjoying a cup of tea is a healthy indulgence that you can enjoy often, and trying different types of teas from different parts of the world is a relaxing and tasty diversion.